The Gestational Diabetes Cookbook

A Meal Plan for a Healthy Pregnancy with Over 40 Easy and Quick Recipes

---

Dr Olivia Tastewell

TABLE OF CONTENTS

INTRODUCTION

JULIET WAS OVERJOYED WHEN SHE FOUND out she was pregnant with her first child. She had always dreamed of becoming a mother and starting a family with her husband. She was determined to do everything right for her baby's health and well-being. But her happiness was soon overshadowed by worry when she learned that she had gestational diabetes, a condition that affects some women during pregnancy and causes high blood sugar levels. She was scared of the possible complications for her and her baby, such as preterm birth, preeclampsia, or birth defects. She felt overwhelmed by the dietary restrictions and lifestyle changes she had to make to manage her condition. She searched for books and online resources to help her cope with gestational diabetes, but she was disappointed by the lack of practical and easy-to-follow advice.

Most of the recipes she found were bland, boring, or complicated. She wanted to enjoy her food and not feel deprived or guilty. She also wanted to save time and money by using simple and affordable ingredients. That's when she discovered the Gestational Diabetes Cookbook, a meal plan for a healthy pregnancy with over 40 easy and quick recipes. This book was written by a registered dietitian and a certified diabetes educator who has helped hundreds of women with gestational diabetes. They understand the challenges and frustrations of living with this condition and offer expert guidance and support.

The Gestational Diabetes Cookbook also features over 40 delicious and nutritious recipes that are easy to make and taste great. You will find recipes for breakfast, lunch, dinner, desserts, and snacks that are suitable for the whole family. These recipes have been meticulously organized in this cookbook.

However, the Gestational Diabetes Cookbook will help you enjoy your pregnancy and nourish your baby without sacrificing your taste buds or your sanity. It will give you the confidence and the tools to manage your condition and have a healthy and happy pregnancy. What are you waiting for? Let's start this wonderful culinary adventure.

Breakfast Recipes

Avocado Toast

Benefits:
- Avocado provides healthy fats and fiber, helping stabilize blood sugar levels.
- Whole-grain toast adds complex carbs for sustained energy.

Ingredients:
- 1 ripe avocado
- 2 slices whole-grain bread
- Salt and pepper to taste

Serving Size: 2
Cooking Time: 5 minutes

Instructions:
1. Toast the whole-grain bread slices.
2. Mash the ripe avocado and spread it evenly on the toast.
3. Season with salt and pepper to taste.

Peanut Butter Rice Cakes

Benefits:
- Peanut butter offers protein and healthy fats.
- Rice cakes provide a low glycemic index option for stable blood sugar.

Ingredients:
- 2 rice cakes
- 2 tablespoons natural peanut butter

Serving Size: 2
Prep Time: 2 minutes

Instructions:
1. Spread peanut butter evenly on each rice cake.

Whole-grain toast with Breakfast Sausages:

- Whole-grain toast offers complex carbs.
- Lean breakfast sausages provide protein without excessive fats.

- 2 slices whole-grain bread
- 4 breakfast sausages
- Cooking spray for sausages

Serving Size: 2
Cooking Time: 10 minutes

1. Toast the whole-grain bread slices.
2. Cook breakfast sausages in a skillet with cooking spray until fully cooked.

Sour Cream Scrambled Eggs

Benefits:
- Eggs offer high-quality protein.
- Sour cream adds creaminess without excessive sugars.

Ingredients:
- 4 eggs
- 2 tablespoons sour cream
- Salt and pepper to taste

Serving Size: 2
Cooking Time: 5 minutes

Instructions:
1. Whisk eggs and sour cream together.
2. Cook scrambled eggs in a non-stick pan over medium heat. Season with salt and pepper.

Greek Yogurt Parfait

Benefits:
- Greek yogurt gives you protein and has good bacteria for your gut.
- Fresh fruits add natural sweetness and fiber.

Ingredients:
- 1 cup Greek yogurt
- 1/2 cup granola
- 1/2 cup mixed berries (strawberries, blueberries)

Serving Size: 1
Cooking Time: 0 minutes

Instructions:
1. In a glass or bowl, layer Greek yogurt, granola, and mixed berries.

Yogurt with a blend of mixed berries

Benefits:
- Greek yogurt offers protein and probiotics.
- Mixed berries add natural sweetness and fiber without causing rapid blood sugar spikes.

Ingredients:
- 1 cup Greek yogurt
- 1/2 cup mixed berries (strawberries, blueberries)

Serving Size: 1
Cooking Time: 0 minutes

Instructions:
1. In a bowl, mix Greek yogurt and top with mixed berries.

Greek Yogurt, Sliced Banana, and Chia Seeds

- Greek yogurt provides protein and probiotics.
- Bananas offer natural sweetness and potassium.
- Chia seeds add fiber and healthy fats.

- 1 cup Greek yogurt
- 1 medium banana, sliced
- 1 tablespoon chia seeds

Serving Size: 1

1. In a bowl, layer Greek yogurt, and sliced banana, and sprinkle with chia seeds.

Boiled Egg with a Slice of Whole-grain Toast

Benefits:
- Boiled eggs provide high-quality protein.
- Whole-grain toast offers complex carbs for sustained energy.

Ingredients:
- 1 boiled egg
- 1 slice whole-grain bread

Serving Size: 1
Cooking Time: 10 minutes

Instructions:
1. Boil an egg to your desired doneness.
2. Toast a slice of whole-grain bread and serve with the boiled egg.

Green Smoothie

Benefits:
- Green leafy vegetables provide essential nutrients.
- Fruits offer natural sweetness and fiber.
- Smoothies allow easy consumption of a variety of ingredients.

Ingredients:
- 1 cup spinach leaves
- 1/2 cucumber, peeled and sliced
- 1/2 banana
- 1/2 cup pineapple chunks
- 1 cup water or unsweetened almond milk
- Ice cubes (optional)

Serving Size: 1
Cooking Time: 5 minutes

Instructions:

1. Blend spinach, cucumber, banana, pineapple, and water (or almond milk) until smooth.
2. If you want, you can put ice cubes in and blend it once more.

Scrambled Eggs with Mushrooms and Spinach

Benefits:
- Eggs provide high-quality protein.
- Mushrooms and spinach add vitamins, minerals, and fiber.

Ingredients:
- 3 eggs
- 1/2 cup sliced mushrooms
- 1 cup fresh spinach
- Salt and pepper to taste

Serving Size: 1
Cooking Time: 10 minutes

Instructions:
1. Whisk eggs and season with salt and pepper.
2. Cook eggs in a pan, adding sliced mushrooms and spinach until fully cooked.

Lunch Recipes

Grilled Chicken Salad

Benefits:
- Grilled chicken provides lean protein.
- Fresh vegetables add essential vitamins and minerals without causing rapid blood sugar spikes.

Ingredients:
- 1 grilled chicken breast, sliced
- Mixed salad greens (lettuce, spinach, arugula)
- Cherry tomatoes, halved
- Cucumber, sliced
- Red bell pepper, sliced
- Balsamic vinaigrette dressing (1 tablespoon)

Serving Size: 1
Cooking Time: 15 minutes (grilling time)

Instructions:
1. Season and grill the chicken breast until fully cooked.
2. In a bowl, combine mixed salad greens, cherry tomatoes, cucumber, and red bell pepper.
3. Top the salad with sliced grilled chicken and drizzle with balsamic vinaigrette.

Veggie Wrap

- Whole-grain wrap provides complex carbs.
- Vegetables offer fiber and essential nutrients.

Ingredients:
- 1 whole-grain wrap
- Hummus (2 tablespoons)
- Mixed vegetables (bell peppers, cucumbers, carrots)
- Spinach leaves

Serving Size: 1
Cooking Time: 5 minutes

Instructions:
1. Spread hummus on the whole-grain wrap.
2. Add a layer of spinach leaves and mixed vegetables.
3. Roll the wrap tightly and slice if desired.

Tuna Salad

Benefits:
- Tuna provides protein and omega-3 fatty acids.
- Including vegetables in your diet provides fiber and important nutrients your body needs.

Ingredients:
- Canned tuna in water (1 can, drained)
- Mixed salad greens
- Cherry tomatoes, halved
- Red onion, finely chopped
- Olive oil (1 tablespoon)
- Lemon juice (1 tablespoon)
- Salt and pepper to taste

Serving Size: 1

Instructions:
1. In a bowl, combine drained tuna, mixed salad greens, cherry tomatoes, and red onion.
2. Add a bit of olive oil and lemon juice, then sprinkle with salt and pepper to taste.

Tuna or Salmon Sandwich

Benefits:
- Tuna or salmon provides protein and omega-3 fatty acids.
- Whole-grain bread offers complex carbs.

Ingredients:
- 1 can tuna or salmon, drained
- 2 slices whole-grain bread
- Lettuce leaves
- Tomato slices
- Mayonnaise (1 tablespoon)

Serving Size: 1

Instructions:
1. Drain tuna or salmon and mix with mayonnaise.
2. Toast the whole-grain bread slices.
3. Assemble the sandwich with lettuce, tomato slices, and the tuna or salmon mixture.

Sesame Ginger Salmon served with Green Beans and Wild Rice

Benefits:
- Wild rice provides complex carbs and fiber.
- Salmon offers protein and omega-3 fatty acids.

Ingredients:
- 1 salmon fillet (6 oz)
- 1 cup green beans, trimmed
- 1/2 cup wild rice, cooked
- Sesame ginger sauce (2 tablespoons)

Serving Size: 1
Cooking Time: 20 minutes

Instructions:
1. Season the salmon with salt and pepper, then grill or bake until fully cooked.
2. Steam or sauté green beans until tender.
3. Serve the salmon over a bed of cooked wild rice and green beans. Drizzle with sesame ginger sauce.

Deconstructed Fajitas

- Lean chicken provides protein.
- Vegetables offer fiber and essential nutrients.

- 1 chicken breast, thinly sliced
- Bell peppers (assorted colors), sliced
- Onion, sliced
- Fajita seasoning (1 tablespoon)
- Whole-grain tortillas (2 small)

Serving Size: 1
Cooking Time: 15 minutes

1. Season chicken with fajita seasoning and cook in a skillet until done.
2. Sauté bell peppers and onions until tender.
3. Serve the sliced chicken, sautéed vegetables, and whole-grain tortillas.

Taco Salad

- Lean ground turkey provides protein.
- Salad greens and vegetables add fiber and nutrients.

Ingredients:
- 1/2 lb lean ground turkey
- Taco seasoning (2 tablespoons)
- Mixed salad greens
- Cherry tomatoes, halved
- Black beans, drained (1/2 cup)
- Avocado, diced
- Salsa (2 tablespoons)

Serving Size: 1
Cooking Time: 15 minutes

Instructions:
1. Cook ground turkey with taco seasoning until fully cooked.
2. In a bowl, layer mixed salad greens, cherry tomatoes, black beans, diced avocado, and seasoned ground turkey.
3. Drizzle with salsa.

Chicken and Lettuce Wrap

Benefits:
- Lean chicken provides protein.
- Lettuce serves as a low-carb alternative to wraps.

Ingredients:
- 1 chicken breast, grilled and sliced
- Large lettuce leaves (such as iceberg or romaine)
- Tomatoes, diced
- Cucumber, julienned
- Greek yogurt sauce (2 tablespoons)

Serving Size: 1
Cooking Time: 15 minutes

Instructions:
1. Grill chicken breast until fully cooked, then slice.
2. Lay out large lettuce leaves and fill with sliced chicken, diced tomatoes, julienned cucumber, and a drizzle of Greek yogurt sauce.

Turkey and Avocado Wrap

Benefits:
- Lean turkey provides protein without excessive fat.
- Avocado offers healthy fats and adds creaminess without spiking blood sugar.

Ingredients:
- 1 whole-grain wrap
- 4 oz lean turkey slices
- 1/2 avocado, sliced
- Lettuce leaves
- Tomato slices
- Greek yogurt or mustard (1 tablespoon, for dressing)

Serving Size: 1

Instructions:
1. Lay out the whole-grain wrap.
2. Arrange turkey slices, avocado, lettuce leaves, and tomato slices.
3. Drizzle with Greek yogurt or spread mustard for added flavor.
4. Roll the wrap tightly and slice if desired.

Quinoa and Black Bean Stuffed Peppers

- Quinoa provides complex carbs and fiber.
- Black beans offer protein and additional fiber.

- 2 bell peppers, halved
- 1 cup cooked quinoa
- 1/2 cup black beans, drained and rinsed
- Onion, finely chopped
- Garlic, minced
- Tomato, diced
- Mexican seasoning blend (cumin, chili powder, paprika - 1 tablespoon)
- Shredded cheese (optional, for topping)

Serving Size: 2
Cooking Time: 30 minutes

1. Preheat the oven to 375°F (190°C).
2. In a pan, sauté onion and garlic until softened. Add cooked quinoa, black beans, diced tomato, and Mexican seasoning.
3. Fill halved bell peppers with the quinoa and black bean mixture.
4. Optional: Top with shredded cheese.

5. Bake in the oven for 20-25 minutes or until peppers are tender.

Dinner Recipes

Asparagus with Grilled Salmon

Benefits:
- Salmon provides protein and omega-3 fatty acids.
- Asparagus is a low-carb vegetable rich in fiber and essential nutrients.

Ingredients:
- 1 salmon fillet (6 oz)
- Fresh asparagus spears (1 bunch)
- Olive oil (1 tablespoon)
- Lemon juice (1 tablespoon)
- Garlic powder, salt, and pepper to taste

Serving Size: 1
Cooking Time: 15 minutes

Instructions:
1. Preheat the grill.
2. Season the salmon with garlic powder, salt, and pepper.
3. Toss asparagus with olive oil, salt, and pepper.
4. Grill salmon and asparagus for about 6-8 minutes per side.
5. Before you serve it, sprinkle some lemon juice on top.

Baked Chicken with Quinoa

- Chicken provides lean protein.
- Quinoa offers complex carbs and fiber.

- 1 chicken breast (6 oz)
- 1/2 cup quinoa, uncooked
- Broccoli florets (1 cup)
- Olive oil (1 tablespoon)
- Lemon zest and juice
- Italian seasoning blend (basil, oregano, thyme
- 1 teaspoon)

Serving Size: 1
Cooking Time: 30 minutes

1. Before you start, heat the oven to 375°F (190°C).
2. Season the chicken breast with lemon zest, Italian seasoning, salt, and pepper.
3. Cook quinoa according to package instructions.
4. Place chicken on a baking sheet, surround with broccoli, and bake for about 20-25 minutes.
5. Serve the baked chicken over a bed of cooked quinoa.

Turkey and Vegetable Stir-fry

Benefits:
- Lean turkey provides protein.
- Including veggies in your meals gives you fiber and important nutrients your body needs.

Ingredients:
- 1/2 lb ground turkey
- Broccoli florets (1 cup)
- Bell peppers (assorted colors), sliced
- Carrots, julienned (1/2 cup)
- Soy sauce (low-sodium - 2 tablespoons)
- Ginger, minced
- Garlic, minced
- Olive oil (1 tablespoon)

Serving Size: 2
Cooking Time: 15 minutes

Instructions:
1. In a pan, heat olive oil and sauté ginger and garlic.
2. Add ground turkey and cook until browned.
3. Stir in broccoli, bell peppers, and julienned carrots.
4. Add soy sauce and cook until vegetables are tender.

Lentil and Vegetable Curry

Benefits:
- Lentils provide plant-based protein and fiber.
- Vegetables add essential nutrients.

Ingredients:
- 1 cup lentils, uncooked
- Mixed vegetables (zucchini, bell peppers, carrots)
- Onion, finely chopped
- Garlic, minced
- Tomato sauce (low-sugar - 1/2 cup)
- Coconut milk (1/2 cup)
- Curry powder, cumin, and coriander (1 tablespoon)

Serving Size: 2
Cooking Time: 40 minutes

Instructions:
1. Cook lentils according to package instructions.
2. In a pan, sauté onion and garlic until softened.
3. Add mixed vegetables and cook until tender.
4. Stir in cooked lentils, tomato sauce, coconut milk, and spices. Simmer until flavors meld.

Beef and Broccoli Stir-fry

- Lean beef provides protein.
- Broccoli is a low-carb vegetable rich in fiber and nutrients.

Ingredients:
- 1/2 lb lean beef strips
- Broccoli florets (1 cup)
- Soy sauce (low-sodium - 2 tablespoons)
- Ginger, minced
- Garlic, minced
- Olive oil (1 tablespoon)

Serving Size: 2
Cooking Time: 15 minutes

Instructions:
1. In a wok or skillet, heat olive oil and sauté ginger and garlic.
2. Add beef strips and cook until browned.
3. Mix in the broccoli and soy sauce, and cook until the broccoli becomes soft.

Zucchini Noodles Prepared with Pesto and Cherry Tomatoes

Benefits:

- this meal provides a low-carb alternative to traditional pasta.
- Pesto adds flavor without excessive sugars.

Ingredients:

- 2 medium-sized zucchinis, spiralized
- Pesto sauce (2 tablespoons)
- Cherry tomatoes, halved (1/2 cup)

Serving Size: 1
Cooking Time: 10 minutes

Instructions:

1. Spiralize zucchinis to create "noodles."
2. In a pan, sauté zucchini noodles until tender.
3. Toss the cooked zucchini noodles with pesto sauce.
4. Place halved cherry tomatoes on the top.

Spaghetti Squash with Turkey Meatballs

Benefits:
- Spaghetti squash is a low-carb alternative to regular pasta.
- Turkey meatballs provide lean protein.

Ingredients:
- 1 spaghetti squash, halved and seeds removed
- Ground turkey (1/2 lb)
- Italian seasoning blend (basil, oregano, thyme - 1 teaspoon)
- Tomato sauce (low-sugar - 1/2 cup)
- Parmesan cheese (optional, for topping)

Serving Size: 2
Cooking Time: 45 minutes

Instructions:
1. Preheat the oven to 375°F (190°C).
2. Roast spaghetti squash halves in the oven for about 30-40 minutes.
3. In a bowl, mix ground turkey with Italian seasoning and form into meatballs.
4. Cook meatballs in a skillet until browned and fully cooked.
5. Scrape the cooked spaghetti squash with a fork to create "spaghetti strands."

6. Top the spaghetti squash with turkey meatballs and tomato sauce. Optional: sprinkle with Parmesan cheese.

Baked Cod with Roasted Vegetables

Benefits:
- Cod is a lean source of protein.
- Roasted vegetables provide essential nutrients.

Ingredients:
- 1 cod fillet (6 oz)
- Assorted vegetables (zucchini, bell peppers, cherry tomatoes)
- Olive oil (1 tablespoon)
- Lemon juice (1 tablespoon)
- Garlic powder, salt, and pepper to taste

Serving Size: 1
Cooking Time: 25 minutes

Instructions:
1. Start by heating the oven to 200°C (400°F).
2. Season the cod fillet with garlic powder, salt, and pepper.
3. Toss vegetables with olive oil and spread them on a baking sheet.
4. Place the seasoned cod on the baking sheet.
5. Bake for about 15-20 minutes or until the cod is cooked through and the vegetables are tender.
6. Drizzle with lemon juice before serving.

Chicken prepared with Vegetable Kebabs

Benefits:
- Chicken provides protein.
- Vegetables offer fiber and essential nutrients.

Ingredients:
- 1 chicken breast, cut into chunks
- Bell peppers (assorted colors), cut into chunks
- Cherry tomatoes
- Red onion, cut into chunks
- Olive oil (1 tablespoon)
- Lemon juice (1 tablespoon)
- Italian seasoning blend (basil, oregano, thyme - 1 teaspoon)

Serving Size: 2
Cooking Time: 20 minutes

Instructions:
1. Preheat the grill or oven.
2. Thread chicken chunks, bell peppers, cherry tomatoes, and red onion onto skewers.
3. Mix olive oil, lemon juice, and Italian seasoning. Brush over kebabs.
4. Grill or bake for about 10-15 minutes or until chicken is fully cooked.

Shrimp and Quinoa Paella

Benefits:
- Shrimp provides protein without excessive fat.
- Quinoa offers complex carbs and fiber.

Ingredients:
- 1/2 lb shrimp, peeled and deveined
- 1 cup quinoa, uncooked
- Bell peppers (assorted colors), diced
- Onion, finely chopped
- Garlic, minced
- Tomato sauce (low-sugar - 1/2 cup)
- Vegetable broth (1 cup)
- Saffron or paprika for flavor (1/2 teaspoon)

Serving Size: 2
Cooking Time: 25 minutes

Instructions:
1. Cook quinoa according to package instructions using vegetable broth for added flavor.
2. In a paella pan or skillet, sauté onion and garlic until softened.
3. Add diced bell peppers and cook until tender.
4. Stir in shrimp, tomato sauce, and saffron or paprika. Cook until the shrimps have become opaque.
5. Serve the shrimp mixture over cooked quinoa.

Smoothies Recipes

Berry Blast

Benefits:
- Berries offer natural sweetness with a lower impact on blood sugar.
- Greek yogurt adds protein and probiotics.

Ingredients:
- 1/2 cup mixed berries (strawberries, blueberries, raspberries)
- 1/2 cup Greek yogurt
- Almond milk (unsweetened - 1/2 cup)
- Chia seeds (1 tablespoon)
- Ice cubes (optional)

Serving Size: 1
Preparation Time: 5 minutes

Instructions:
1. Blend mixed berries, Greek yogurt, almond milk, and chia seeds until smooth.
2. Add ice cubes if you like to make it chilly and blend again.

Green Power

Benefits:
- Leafy greens provide essential nutrients with a low glycemic index.
- Avocado adds healthy fats for satiety.

Ingredients:
- 1 cup spinach leaves
- 1/2 avocado
- Banana
- Almond milk (unsweetened - 1/2 cup)
- Lemon juice (1 tablespoon)

Serving Size: 1
Preparation Time: 5 minutes

Instructions:
1. Blend spinach leaves, avocado, banana, almond milk, and lemon juice until smooth.

Tropical Paradise

Benefits:

- Tropical fruits offer natural sweetness.
- Coconut water hydrates without added sugars.

Ingredients:

- 1/2 cup pineapple chunks
- 1/2 cup mango chunks
- Coconut water (1/2 cup)
- Greek yogurt (2 tablespoons)
- Mint leaves (optional, for garnish)

Serving Size: 1
Preparation Time: 5 minutes

Instructions:

1. Blend pineapple chunks, mango chunks, coconut water, and Greek yogurt until smooth.
2. If you like, you can decorate it with mint leaves.

Berry Spinach

Benefits:
- Berries provide antioxidants and fiber.
- Spinach adds iron and other essential nutrients.

Ingredients:
- 1/2 cup mixed berries (strawberries, blueberries, raspberries)
- Handful of spinach leaves
- Banana
- Almond milk (unsweetened - 1/2 cup)
- Flaxseeds (1 tablespoon)

Serving Size: 1
Preparation Time: 5 minutes

Instructions:
1. Blend mixed berries, spinach leaves, banana, almond milk, and flaxseeds until smooth.

Mango Ginger

- Mango provides natural sweetness.
- Ginger adds flavor and may have anti-inflammatory properties.

Ingredients:
- 1 cup mango chunks
- Greek yogurt (1/2 cup)
- Almond milk (unsweetened - 1/2 cup)
- Fresh ginger, grated (1 teaspoon)
- Turmeric (optional, a pinch)

Serving Size: 1
Preparation Time: 5 minutes

Instructions:
1. Blend mango chunks, Greek yogurt, almond milk, grated ginger, and turmeric until smooth.

Blueberry Almond

- Blueberries offer antioxidants and fiber with a lower impact on blood sugar.
- Almonds add healthy fats and protein for satiety.

Ingredients:
- 1/2 cup blueberries
- Almond butter (1 tablespoon)
- Greek yogurt (1/2 cup)
- Almond milk (unsweetened - 1/2 cup)
- Chia seeds (1 tablespoon)

Serving Size: 1
Preparation Time: 5 minutes

Instructions:
1. Blend blueberries, almond butter, Greek yogurt, almond milk, and chia seeds until smooth.

Peachy Green

Benefits:
- Peaches provide natural sweetness without excessive sugars.
- Leafy greens add essential nutrients with a low glycemic index.

Ingredients:
- 1 cup sliced peaches
- Handful of spinach leaves
- Banana
- Coconut water (1/2 cup)
- Mint leaves (optional, for garnish)

Serving Size: 1
Preparation Time: 5 minutes

Instructions:
1. Blend sliced peaches, spinach leaves, nanas, and coconut water until smooth.
2. Garnish with mint leaves if desired.

Raspberry Coconut

Benefits:

- Raspberries offer antioxidants and fiber.
- Coconut milk adds creaminess without added sugars.

Ingredients:

- 1/2 cup raspberries
- Coconut milk (1/2 cup)
- Greek yogurt (1/2 cup)
- Honey (optional, for sweetness)
- Shredded coconut (optional, for garnish)

Serving Size: 1
Preparation Time: 5 minutes

Instructions:

1. Blend raspberries, coconut milk, Greek yogurt, and honey until smooth.
2. If you like, you can decorate it with shredded coconut.

Pineapple Kale

Benefits:

- Pineapple provides natural sweetness.
- Kale adds iron and other essential nutrients.

Ingredients:

- Pineapple chunks (1 cup)

- Handful of kale leaves (stems removed)
- Banana
- Almond milk (unsweetened - 1/2 cup)
- Flaxseeds (1 tablespoon)

Serving Size: 1
Preparation Time: 5 minutes

Instructions:
1. Blend pineapple chunks, kale leaves, banana, almond milk, and flaxseeds until smooth.

Chocolate Banana

Benefits:
- Bananas provide natural sweetness.
- Cocoa powder adds chocolate flavor without added sugars.

Ingredients:
- Banana
- Cocoa powder (1 tablespoon)
- Greek yogurt (1/2 cup)
- Almond milk (unsweetened - 1/2 cup)
- Peanut butter (1 tablespoon)

Serving Size: 1
Preparation Time: 5 minutes

Instructions:
1. Blend banana, cocoa powder, Greek yogurt, almond milk, and peanut butter until smooth.

Meal plan

Day 1:
- Breakfast: Berry Blast
- Lunch: Grilled Chicken Salad
- Dinner: Grilled Salmon with Asparagus

Day 2:
- Breakfast: Green Power Smoothie
- Lunch: Veggie Wrap
- Dinner: Baked Chicken with Quinoa

Day 3:
- Breakfast: Tropical Paradise Smoothie
- Lunch: Tuna Salad
- Dinner: Turkey and Vegetable Stir-fry

Day 4:
- Breakfast: Berry Spinach Smoothie
- Lunch: Tuna or Salmon Sandwich
- Dinner: Lentil and Vegetable Curry

Day 5:
- Breakfast: Mango Ginger Smoothie
- Lunch: Green Beans and Wild Rice with Sesame Ginger Salmon
- Dinner: Beef and Broccoli Stir-fry

Day 6:
- Breakfast: Blueberry Almond Smoothie
- Lunch: Deconstructed Fajitas
- Dinner: Zucchini Noodles with Pesto and Cherry Tomatoes

Day 7:
- Breakfast: Peachy Green Smoothie
- Lunch: Taco Salad
- Dinner: Spaghetti Squash with Turkey Meatballs

CONCLUSION

In conclusion, **the Gestational Diabetes Cookbook** serves as a comprehensive guide to maintaining optimal nutrition during pregnancy. As we embarked on this culinary journey, our primary goal was to provide expectant mothers with flavorful and nutritious meal options that specifically cater to the challenges of gestational diabetes. Throughout these pages, we've curated a diverse collection of over 40 easy and quick recipes, each thoughtfully crafted to support both the well-being of the mother and the development of the baby. From a vibrant breakfast to a satisfying lunch and delightful dinner with some smoothies, this cookbook offers a wealth of delicious choices that adhere to dietary guidelines for gestational diabetes management.

Our emphasis on simplicity ensures that these recipes are not only health-conscious but also practical for the busy lifestyles of expectant mothers. By incorporating wholesome ingredients and mindful preparation, we aim to empower readers to make informed and nourishing food choices throughout their pregnancy journey.

May this cookbook be a source of inspiration and culinary joy, proving that a gestational diabetes-friendly meal plan can be both satisfying and delicious. Wishing you a healthy and vibrant pregnancy filled with flavorful moments at the table.